Yoga For Men

*Top 30 Illustrated Poses for
a Stronger Body and a Sharper Mind*

Copyright © 2015 by Tai Morello

Table of Contents

Introduction 1

What is Yoga? 2

Why Every Man Should do Yoga 4

Yoga Poses to build strength and flexibility 6

Yoga Poses for cognitive benefits and psychological health ... 35

Yoga Poses for Meditation 39

How to Meditate 45

The Benefits of Yoga 47

Turning Yoga into a habit 49

Conclusion 52

Bonus: Free Guided Meditation Series (5 Audiobooks) 53

Preview of The Meditation Beginner's Bible 54

Preview of The Mindfulness Beginner's Bible 62

Introduction

If you think yoga isn't for men, just take a look at basketball stars Blake Griffin and Dirk Nowitzki. They are just two of the big names that have trained with renowned yoga coach Kent Katich to improve their physical and mental strength, flexibility, balance and prevent injuries. If you're looking to build a stronger, more toned body while sharpening your mind, then yoga perfect for you.

From the outside, yoga can seem like an esoteric, mystical endeavor exclusively reserved to Tibetan monks and spiritual adepts. This could not be further from the truth. Yoga is not only accessible to anyone, it is easy to learn if you have the right mindset and the benefits are only a few minutes away.

In fact, several studies have confirmed that a single yoga class for inpatients at a psychiatric hospital had the ability to significantly reduce tension, anxiety, depression, anger, hostility, and fatigue.

In this book you will learn why many highly successful men like Lebron James Jr, Jay Cutler and Blake Griffin set aside time off their busy schedules to engage in the life-changing practice of yoga.

This book will show you how to instill simple yoga techniques into your daily routine, inevitably leading you to a healthier and stronger body and mind. You will discover how yoga can have profound effects not just on your body, but on virtually every aspect of your life – your mind, relationships, health and even your career.

What is Yoga?

Before we get into the practical how-to of various yogic poses, we should consider what it is we're actually talking about and what it's for. Yoga has been practiced in India for thousands of years. The word *yoga* comes from Sanskrit and is related to the English word *yoke*. Just as a yoke joins an ox to a cart or a plow, *yoga* joins mind and body together in a well-integrated union. On a spiritual level, yoga unites the individual's personal experience to an experience of the absolute reality.

Yoga refers to a broad variety of ancient Indian spiritual practices. These practices are designed to liberate the individual from their ordinary, bound, unfree experience of the self and the world, into an expansive, unlimited state of complete freedom.

So right away we can do away with the idea that, in order to do yoga, you need to sign up with a religious group and give up your own beliefs, adopting a new set of doctrines and strange behaviors. If you're not into the metaphysical ideas behind yoga as spiritual transformation, that's no problem. Yoga is, first and foremost, *personal, practical,* and *experiential.* What you get out of it depends on what you bring into it; your goals and purposes for doing yoga will determine what kind of positive effect it has on your life.

In particular, the popular perception associates yoga with a system of bendy, twisty physical movements and positions. Some may even think yoga is just glorified stretching. But yoga is about more than just stretching. It's about creating balance in body and mind, and joining the two together and bringing them into close communication.

Recent scientific research into the effects of yoga on the body and mind have shown that these physical practices have enormous benefits for physical and psychological health. They can help you lose weight, tone muscles, treat a number of medical problems, improve your flexibility and posture, keep your muscles relaxed and supple, regulate your appetite, etc. They also decrease the all-too-common psychological sufferings of stress, anxiety, and depression, improve concentration and mindfulness, and boost your mood and brainpower overall.

Yoga offers a profound sense of physical and psychological wellbeing. Through the practice of yoga, your body and mind will become more and more closely integrated. That's the central lesson of yoga: by connecting with our bodies more deeply, we go further into our experience as embodied beings in the world. That, in turn, will enrich our lives, as we bring the mindful awareness of yoga into our everyday world.

Finally, a word of warning needs to be said about the practices that follow. Some yoga poses can be dangerous if you're not careful. You can get injured trying to get into some positions. So proceed with caution. Always pay attention to what your body is telling you, and don't do anything if it starts to feel uncomfortable or painful. Sometimes your body will whisper, "Um, maybe not." Sometimes it will scream, "NO WAY, STOP NOW!" Be careful and sensitive to these messages.

While this book is intended to give you an introduction to the physical poses and the meditative side of yoga, it's strongly advised that you learn yoga under the guidance of a qualified and experienced instructor. A good yoga teacher can help you avoid mistakes and injury, correct your posture, and guide you into more advanced stages of practice as you get deeper and deeper into yoga.

Why Every Man Should do Yoga

Believe it or not, yoga was created by men and for men. Some ancient yoga manuals go as far as advising yogis to avoid women in order to remain focused and pure.

Most yoga lineages were started by men and practiced only by men. Yoga poses are specifically designed to strengthen and open every muscle in the body. While machines at your gym target one muscle or muscle group with no improvement in mobility, every yoga sequence improves both strength and mobility for several muscles at once.

In downward dog for instance, which is covered later in the book, the calves are being elongated while the shoulders are strengthened as they hold the body up. At the same time, the lower back is stretched, which relieves tension. The core is also solicited by pulling the bellybutton to the spine! There probably isn't a single machine in your gym that can do all of that.

Granted, twenty first century Yoga is female. When you look around the classes, you'll see women massively outnumber men. But the truth is yoga isn't just for flexible ladies in tight clothes. Besides allow you to meet flexible women, Yoga can help you build a basis for weightlifting, cut belly fat, hone your mental focus and rid your system of toxins.

Here are 6 reasons why every man should practice Yoga:

Yoga widens your range of motion
Practicing yoga increases your range of motion and allows access to more muscle fiber, resulting in greater muscle hypertrophy. So if you are lifting weights, yoga will make you even stronger as you'll be able to activate ignored sections of

muscle. Renowned Bodybuilder Jay Cutler has used Yoga to stretch his pectorals even further, and in turn build more muscle mass in his chest.

Deep abdominal breathing
Many Yoga poses require you to breathe deeply into your stomach. This activates the parasympathetic nervous systems, lowers cortisol, which is a hormone that makes your body hold on to belly fat. Breathing deeply will drastically reduce the amount of stress in your daily life.

Lower Heart Rate
Over time, yoga routines will challenge your heart, improve your breathing rate and strengthen your cardiovascular system. This will lead to a lower overall heart rate, a better breathing volume and more oxygen in your body.

Yoga works the entire body
Doing yoga will build strength in muscles you never even knew you had. Yoga solicits the strength of your entire body in most poses, which over time will help you sculpt a stronger, more chiseled and toned body.

Yoga can increase your libido
Practicing yoga increases blood flow to the groin, which will help you perform better in the bedroom. The relaxation and concentration that yoga brings can be translated into a better sex life by helping you channel your sexual energy, lasting longer and being more responsive to your partner.

Yoga helps you smell better
No joke. Michael Hewitt, who founded Sarva Yoga Academy says: "Pheromonally, regular practice is more effective than cologne." Yoga helps remove toxins as you sweat and exhale, which makes your sweat smell sweeter.

Yoga Poses to build strength and flexibility

Remember that when you're just getting started, 10 minutes of yoga is enough. When you're just getting started, pick three to five poses that you are comfortable with and practice them each day. As a general guideline you can aim to hold each pose for 30 seconds to a minute. Over time, your flexibility will increase and you'll be able to do even the most challenging poses.

1. Adho Mukha Svanasana / Downward-Facing Dog

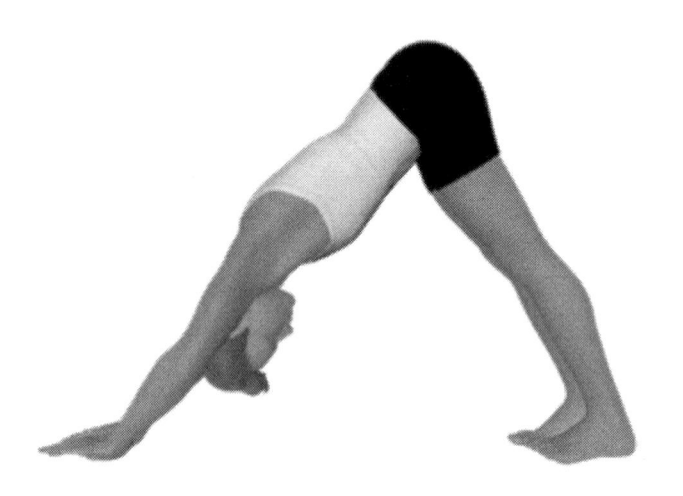

Straighten your arms and legs and push your butt up towards the ceiling. Lower your head between your arms, so that your ears are aligned with your inner arm. Press the heels of your feet to the floor. Take some time to breathe deeply and let yourself feel the stretch in your calves, thighs, shoulders, and arms.

It is important not to force yourself into position, so as to avoid injury. Get your body as close as it can comfortably get into downward-facing dog, and no closer.

Benefits: One of the most important poses for men. It stretches and strengthens the legs, arms, shoulders, and spine. By pressing the heels to the ground, you stretch the calf muscles, which can benefit conditions such as tendinitis of the foot. It improves digestion and the immune system and stimulates circulation. The downward position of the head increases blood flow to the sinuses. It also energizes the body and mind and helps reduce stress. It's great for back pain and tight shoulders. If you can only do one pose a day, start with downward-facing dog.

Contraindications: Injury to the back, hips, arms or shoulders. High blood pressure.

2. Utthita Ashwa Sanchalanasana / High Lunge Pose

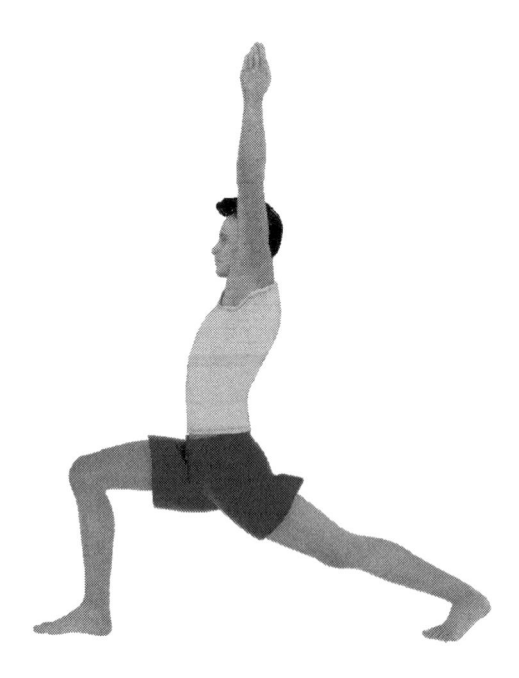

From downward-facing dog, round your right knee toward your nose. Then step your right foot between your hands and transfer your weight into your feet. Finally, reach your arms toward the ceiling, framing your face. Only the ball of your left foot should touch the ground and your toes should point directly forward. Make sure your right knee is bent at a 90° angle and keep it in a fixed position.

Benefits: High lunge opens the hips and chest, stretches the groin and legs, lengthens the spine and builds strength in the lower body.

Contraindications: Recent or chronic injury to the legs or hips.

Virabhadrasana I / Warrior One Pose

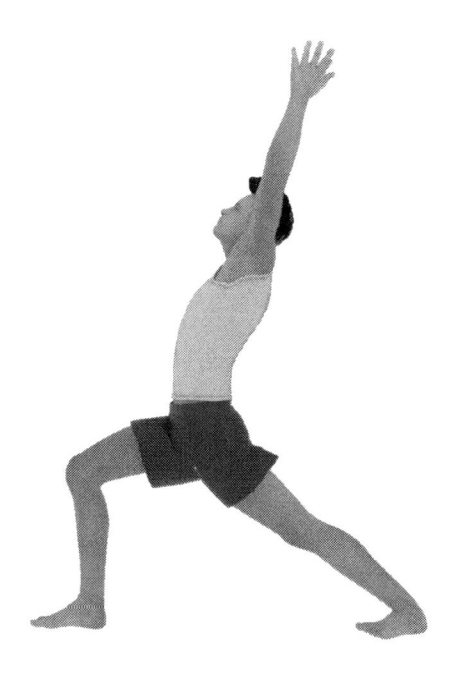

From High Lunge, use arms to slightly draw back the torso. Ensure sure the right knee is directly over the right ankle. Draw the shoulders towards the spine to open the chest. In warrior one, your left foot is flat on the ground at a 45° angle to the left.

Benefits: Warrior one stretches men in two important areas – the hips and shoulders. It is also a strengthening posture for the thighs and knees which builds resilience for joints during running or other high impact sports. Warrior one can make your shoulders more powerful.

30 Tadasana / Mountain pose

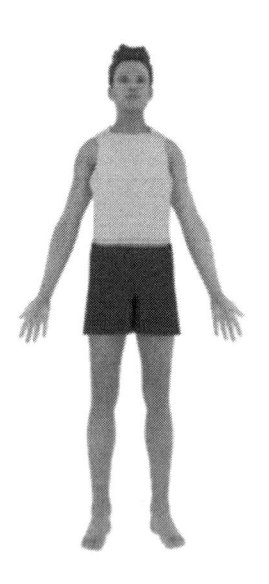

The mountain pose may look simple, but it's incredibly powerful. Stand with your toes touching the floor and your heels slightly apart. Distribute your weight evenly on the entire surface of your feet. Flex your calf and quadriceps muscles. Solicit your core muscles and open your chest by drawing your shoulders back and down. Point your hands toward the floor, lengthen your neck and lift your chin slightly. Now breathe deeply.

Benefits: The mountain pose will make more grounded and more centered as a man. It's a confident posture that affects your psychology as it conveys power and confidence. It also builds strength in the legs, glutes, core, arms, and back.

6 Virabhadrasana II / Warrior Two Pose

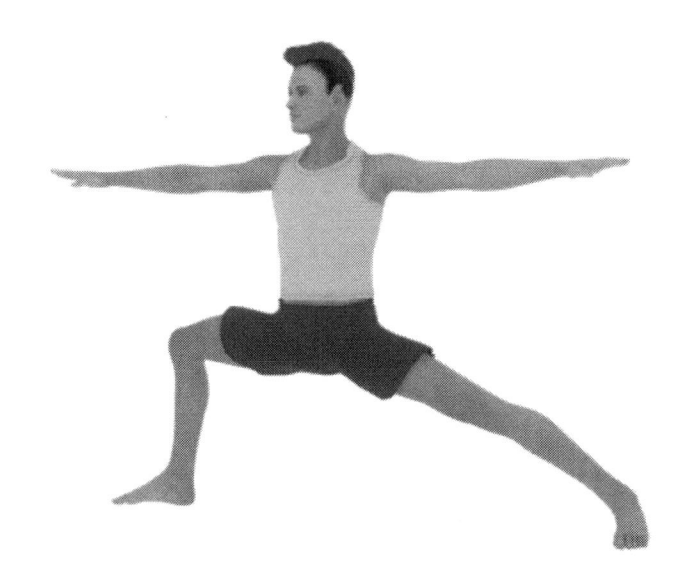

From the Mountain Pose, step your feet about 4 feet apart. Raise your arms to the sides and turn your right foot slightly to the right and your left foot 90° to the left. Make sure your heels are aligned. Turn your left thigh outward and bend your left knee over the left ankle, making the shin perpendicular to the floor.

Avoid leaning your torso over the left thigh, turn your head to the left and look over your fingers

Benefits: Warrior II builds strength in the legs and opens the hips and chest. It develops concentration, balance and groundedness. It improves circulation, respiration and energizes the entire body.

Utkatasana / Chair pose

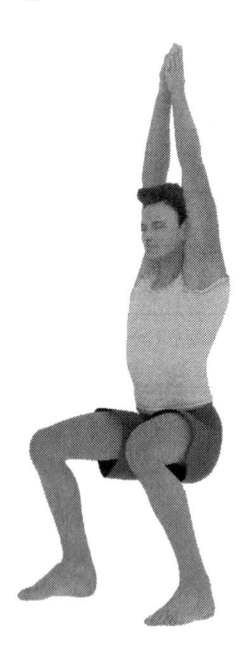

From the Mountain pose, inhale and slowly bring your arms above your head, perpendicular to the floor. Then, exhale as you bend your knees so as to make your thighs parallel to the floor. Draw your shoulders back and reach your elbows towards your ears. Shift your weight toward your heels so that you could easily lift your toes. Breathe deeply and smoothly.

Benefits: The chair pose is a powerful pose that tones the entire body, particularly the thighs. It also helps develop more stability.

Contraindications: Headaches, low blood pressure, insomnia.

3. Phalakasana / Plank Pose

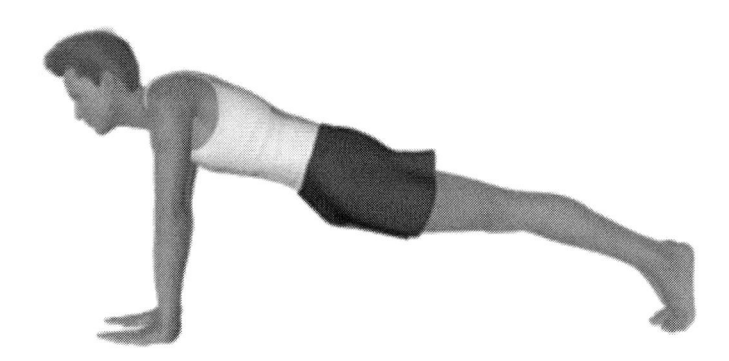

Start by kneeling on the floor, then raise your buttocks so that your thighs are vertical. Lean forward and put your hands on the floor, palms down, beneath your shoulders and at shoulders width. Lift the buttocks up, keeping your knees straight, so that you are balancing on your hands and toes. Keep your buttocks slightly lifted, against the force of gravity that pulls your hips towards the floor and arches your back. Keep your back straight, your neck aligned with your spine so that the eyes are looking towards the floor.

In the final position, you should feel that the muscles in both your back and abdomen are engaged. Maintain this for as long as you can. You may even find that your body starts shaking while you hold this position. If it's too difficult to support the weight on your hands, try lowering yourself on your elbows.

As a variation, from the final position, try lifting each leg alternately until it's parallel to the floor and the weight is distributed to the other foot.

Benefits: Plank pose tones the abdominal and back muscles. It strengthens the arms, shoulders, and wrists. It improves balance.

Vasishtasana / Side Plank Pose

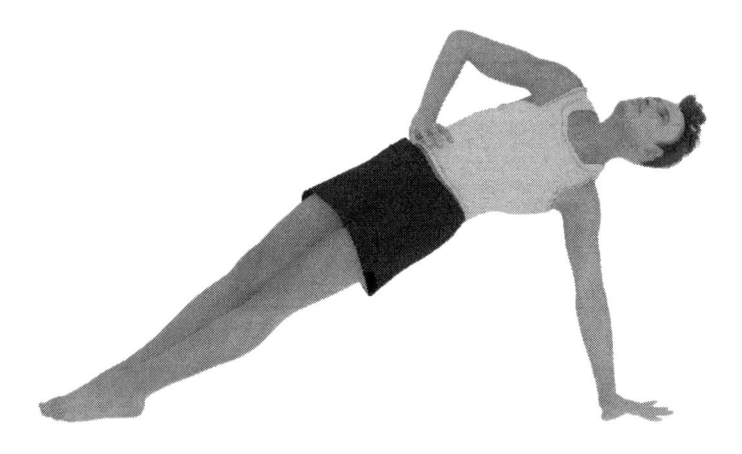

From plank pose, shift onto the side of your right foot, so that your right foot and right hand support the entire weight of your body. Your left foot rests on your right, and the left hand rests on the left hip.

The right arm should not be directly below the shoulder, but a little higher. Keep your back straight, so that your spine is aligned with your legs. Breathe normally.

Alternately, you may find it easier to support your weight on your elbow instead of your hand. In other variations, lift your left arm so that it is vertical. You may also lift your left leg, or even try to hold your left foot with your left hand, while keeping both leg and arm straight.

Perform this pose three times on each side, right and left.

Benefits: Side plank pose strengthens and tones the arms, legs, and lower back, as well as the abdomen. In particular, it targets the oblique muscles, reducing the appearance of love handles.

7. Bhujangasana / Cobra Pose

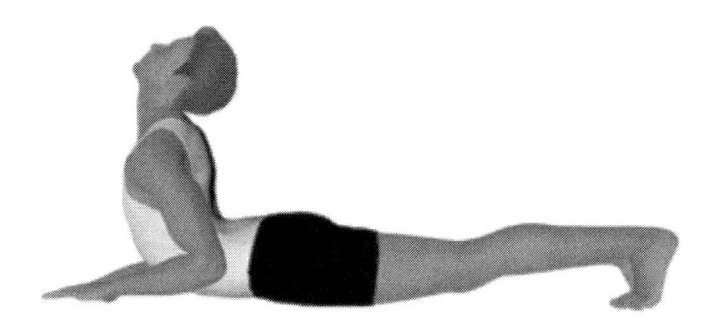

Lower your hips to the floor. As you inhale, straighten your arms somewhat but keep them slightly bent. Arch your back and lift your chest from the floor. Bend your head back, gazing upwards with your eyes. Only lift your chest and arch your back as far as they can go without lifting your hips and pelvic area from the floor; unless your spine is very flexible, your elbows will probably remain somewhat bent. The feet may be either lie flat on the floor, or balance on bent toes. Squeeze your buttocks to remove pressure from your lower back.

Benefits: Cobra pose increases flexibility in the spine, helping to relieve stiffness in the lower back especially. It stretches the muscles in your chest and abdomen. It stimulates abdominal organs, in particular improving digestion and helping to alleviate constipation. It elevates your mood and relieves stress. For women, it helps promote regular menstruation.

Contraindications: If you have spinal problems or pain in your back, you may find this position a bit uncomfortable or painful, so don't try to force yourself into it. Take it easy on spine, keeping your elbows bent, and do not arch your back to the point of discomfort.

8 Uttanasana / Standing forward bend Pose

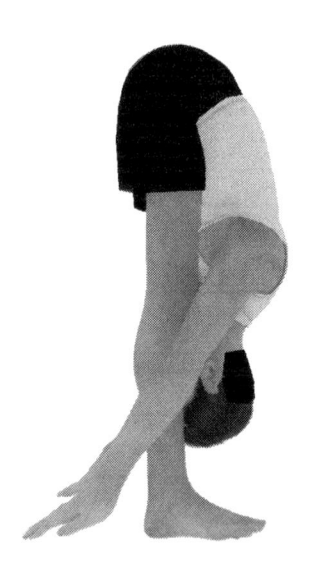

Stand with your feet together and fold your torso over your legs. (Use your hip joints to bend over) Then, place your hands next to your feet or on the ground in front of you. Inhale slowly and extend your chest to stretch your spine.

Benefits: Stretches the hamstrings, back and muscles of the spine. Also calms the mind.

Contraindications: Recent or chronic injury to the legs, hips, back or shoulders.

12 Urdhva mukha svanasana / Upward facing dog

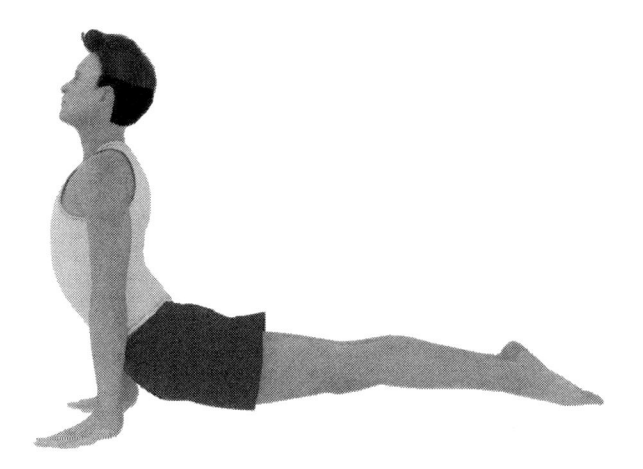

Begin by lying on the floor in prone position. Bend your elbows and put your palms on the floor beside your waist. Make sure your forearms are perpendicular to the floor. As you inhale, press your hands into the floor toward the back, as if you were pushing yourself forward. Then, bring your torso up and lift your legs slightly as you exhale. Finally, draw your shoulders back and look straight ahead.

Benefits: Upward-facing dog opens the chest and builds strength in the back and arms. If you sit behind a desk all day long, this pose will help you by opening the abdomen and hips. It's also a great warm up before a more demanding form of exercise.

Naukasana / Boat Pose

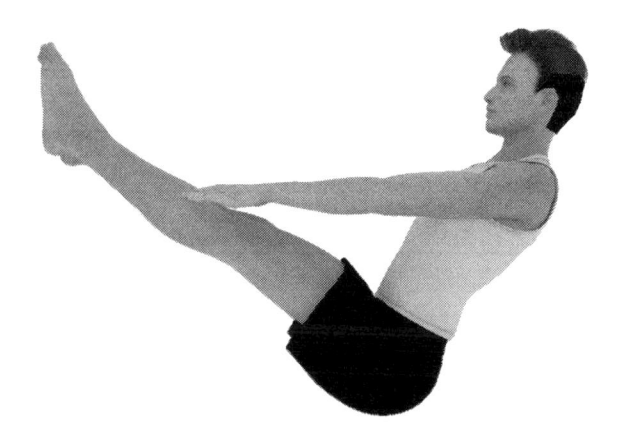

Boat pose is meant to be performed from a supine (lying down) position, and is best performed together with other supine postures. From the supine position, breathe in, then hold the breath as you raise your legs and trunk, together with the shoulders and head, from the ground. Hold the arms straight and parallel to the ground, palms facing down. The whole body should form the shape of a triangle pointing downwards, balanced on the buttocks. Keep your spine straight and gaze at your feet.

Hold this position without breathing for as long as you can—basically, until you need to breathe again. As you return to a supine position (*lie down on your back*), breathe out again. Allow all the muscles in your body to relax. Then repeat four times, for a total of five rounds.

Benefits: Boat pose exercises your core, especially strengthening and toning the abdominal muscles and helping to remove excess belly fat. It also strengthens and tones muscles in the shoulders, arms, and thighs. It benefits and improves the function of abdominal organs.

14 Badhakonasana / Butterfly pose

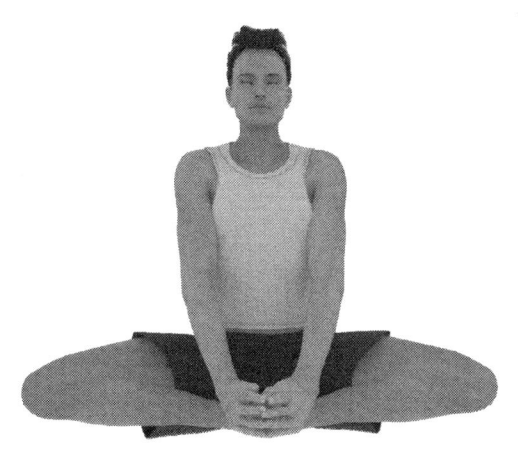

Begin by sitting with your spine straight and legs spread straight out. Then, bend your knees and bring your feet close to your pelvic area. Make sure the soles of your feet touch each other.

Now grab your feet with your hands, placing them under your feet to support them. Inhale slowly and deeply. Then exhale as you bring your thighs and knees toward the floor.

Start flapping your legs up and down like a butterfly. Begin slowly and gradually increase the speed. Keep breathing normally. Fly as fast as you comfortably can, then slow down gradually until you stop completely.

Push your knees and thighs toward the floor by using your elbows. Breathe deeply as you feel the stretch in your inner thighs. As you exhale, slowly release the posture, straighten the legs in front of you and relax.

Benefits: Increases blood flow to the pelvis, prostate, bladder and kidneys. Improves sexual performance.

Contraindications: Groin or knee injury.

15 Ardha Kapotasana / Half pigeon

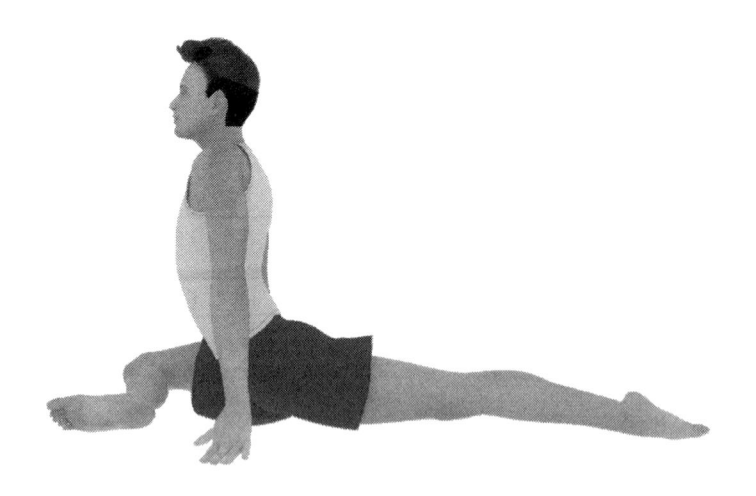

Begin by kneeling on the floor. Bring your left leg behind you. Bend your right knee so that your right foot is close to your left pelvic bone. Place your fingers on the ground for balance and look in front of you.

Benefits: Half Pigeon is a great pose for tight hips. It can be difficult to maintain at first, but over time it will become easier as you open your hips more and more. It will help you in any physical activity, including carrying heavy objects.

Setu Asana / Bridge Pose

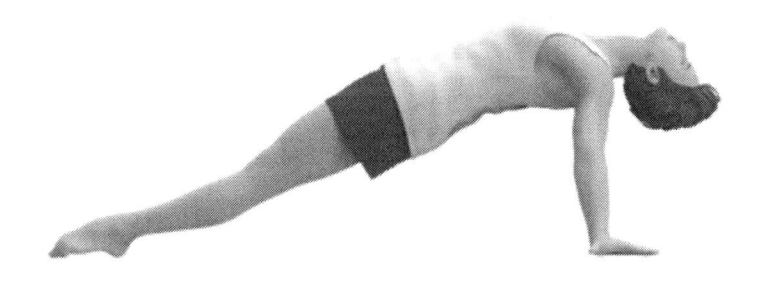

Sit on the floor with your legs extended in front of you. Place your hands, fingers pointing backwards, on the floor about one foot behind you. Keep your elbows straight. You should be leaning backwards slightly.

Inhale, then, holding the breath, lift your waist and torso, so that your feet and hands are touching the ground and the rest of your body is arching upwards. Ideally, the feet should rest flat against the floor. Relax your neck and allow your head to hang loosely.

Hold the position for as long as you are comfortable, then exhale and gently lower your body to the original seated position.

This can be repeated for ten rounds.

Benefits: Bridge pose strengthens and tones the lower back muscles. It also strengthens the arms and legs. It benefits posture, back problems, and stretches the achilles tendon.

Ustrasana / Camel Pose

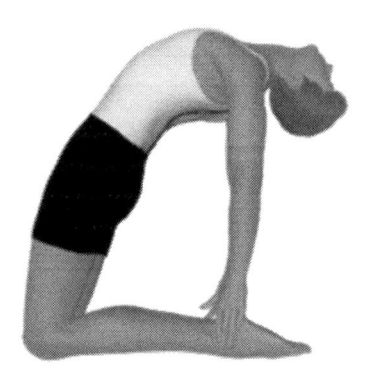

Kneel down on your knees, keeping them hips-width apart, with your back straight and arms hanging by your sides. Keep your feet and knees together. Lean back and grasp one heel with one hand, then the other heel with the other hand. Thrust your stomach forward while keeping your thighs perpendicular to the floor. Arch your back and neck, and bring the head back until you're gazing at the ceiling. Allow some of the weight to fall on your arms and some on your legs, so that the arms support the upper back. Breathe shallowly while in camel pose.

If you're a beginner, you might find it difficult to get into this position. It's worth repeating: Don't force yourself. You might find it easier if you rest on the balls of the feet instead of extending them so that they lie flat on the floor.

Benefits: Camel pose deeply stretches all the muscles in the front of the body, including the neck, chest, abs, thighs, and groin. It is an especially good stretch for the hip flexors. It's also excellent for strengthening the back and improving posture. By stretching the abdominal muscles, it also improves digestion.

Contraindications: Do not try camel pose if you suffer from serious back problems or high blood pressure.

Ardha Halasana / Half Plough Pose

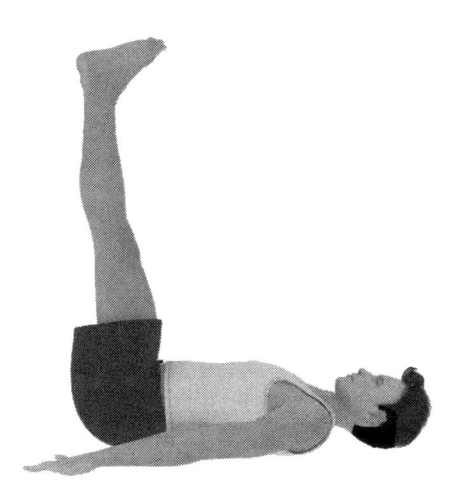

Lie on the back in the supine position with your legs together. While inhaling, left both legs up slowly until they are at a right angle to the floor. Don't lift the buttocks from the floor, but keep them and the back lying flat against the floor. Your abs should be doing the work in this position. Hold this position, and your breath, for several seconds. Then exhale and gently lower your legs to the floor.

That completes one round. It should be repeated for five to ten rounds.

Alternately, you can bring your legs to a forty-five degree angle to your torso. In either case, with your legs held at ninety or forty-five degrees, you can experiment with separating them and bring them back together, and other movements, to reach different abdominal muscles.

Benefits: Half plough pose engages and tones abdominal muscles, removes belly fat, and helps you get closer to achieving a six-pack. It tones the muscles in the thighs and hips, as well. It improves digestion and flatulence.

Dhanurasana / Bow Pose

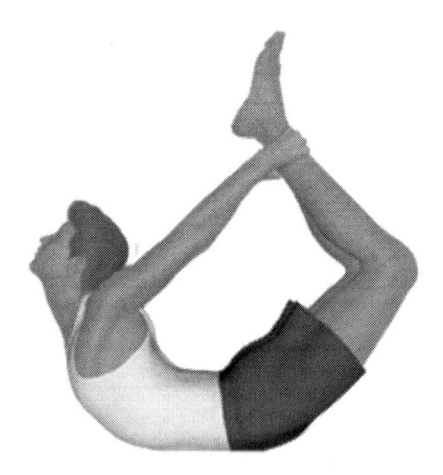

Lie on your stomach with your chin on the floor and your feet hips-width apart. Bend your knees and bring the heels as close as you can to your buttocks. Grasp the ankles with your hands, and, keeping your arms straight, extend the legs so that your chest and knees lift from the floor and the feet move upwards, away from the body. Your abdomen and groin should remain on the floor. Arch your neck so that your eyes are directed upwards. Your legs should be doing the work to hold you in position, allowing the rest of your muscles—back, abs, chest, arm—to relax.

Continue holding this position and breathing for about twenty seconds. Then exhale and gently relax the leg muscles, slowly lowering yourself to the floor. Complete about five rounds.

Benefits: Bow pose strengthens the back and abs and tones muscles in the legs, arms, and chest. It improves your flexibility and decreases stress.

Tadasana / Palm Tree Pose

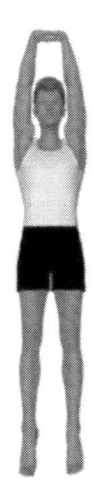

Stand with your feet together or slightly apart and find your balance, arms hanging loosely by your side. Raise your arms overhead and interlock your fingers, turning your palms upward so they face the ceiling. Then lower your hands until your knuckles are resting on the top of our head.

Look forward at a fixed point in front of you and do not move your gaze from this spot. As you inhale, stretch your arms high above you, pulling your shoulder and chest upward with them. Push yourself up on tiptoes, and stretch the whole body in that position, maintaining balance and stability while holding your breath for a few moments.

Then lower the heels and bring your hands back down to their resting position on top of your head, while exhaling. Do five or more rounds, taking a few moments to rest between each round.

Benefits: Palm tree pose stretches the spinal column and can even increase your height. It strengthens muscles in the core, toning the abdominal and back muscles and improving the overall balance of the body. It also strengthens and tones muscles in the arms and legs.

For a variation of this position, once you have achieved good stability and balance in *tadasana,* try taking four steps forward and backward while balancing on your toes.

Tiryana Tadasana / Swaying Palm Tree Pose

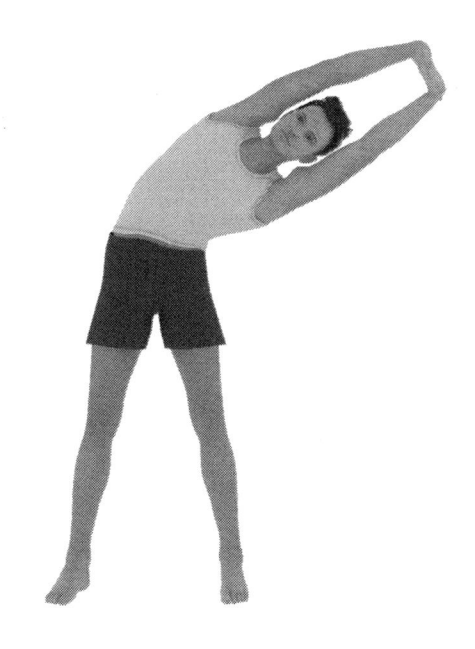

Stand with your feet about two feet apart. With your arms lowered, interlock your fingers and turn the palms outward. As you inhale, raise the arms above your head, as in *tadasana*. Then exhale and bend the body to the left without twisting your abdomen or moving forward or backward. Hold the breath for a few seconds without inhaling. Then, as you straighten out and resume the upright position, breathe in again.

Now repeat the bending movement, only this time bend the body to the right side while exhaling. Again hold that position for a few seconds without breathing in. Then inhale again as you resume a straightened position. Finally, exhale as you lower your arms again. Rest for a moment. Then perform several more rounds, as many as five to ten in total.

Benefits: Swaying palm tree pose strengthens the oblique muscles, toning them and removing love handles. It engages the hard-to-reach muscles that cover the rib cage. It adds overall balance to your core, improving the stability of your posture. It also stretches the spine, relieving minor back injuries such as slipped disc. It also stimulates digestion and relieves constipation.

Once you have stability and flexibility with this posture, you can try doing it while standing on your toes as in *tadasana*.

Kati Chakrasana / Waist-Rotating Pose

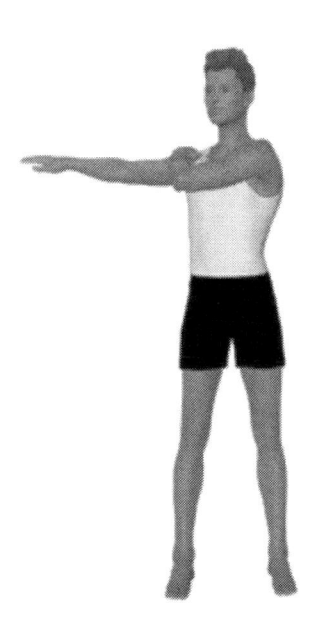

Stand with your feet about one and a half feet apart, with your arms by your side. As you inhale, raise your arms up so that they spread out on either side of you, parallel to the floor. Then, while exhaling, twist your torso around to your left, bringing your right hand to rest on your left shoulder and wrapping your left arm all the away around the back so that the left hand rests on the right waist. Twist your head as far to the left as you can without straining, taking care to make sure that your neck and posture are straight and upright. Hold the breath for several seconds, stretching your abdomen and allowing the muscles to relax. Don't allow your feet to lift from the ground while twisting.

Then inhale as you resume the initial position, and repeat the twist, this time turning to your right. Again hold the breath, and again inhale as you resume the initial position.

Complete at least five rounds. The movements should be performed smoothly, without any sudden movements or jerkiness. For more of a workout, twist left and right at a faster pace.

Benefits: Waist-rotating pose stretches and tones the muscles in the waist, back, and hips. It also loosens up the arms and shoulders. Taken together with palm tree pose and swaying palm tree pose, waist-rotating pose forms the third part of a sequence that can be performed at any time of the day when one is feeling tired or stiff. This threefold sequence is especially useful for office workers who have to sit for long hours, as it loosens up the spine, elevates depressed mood, alleviates stress, and infuses your body and mind with extra energy.

26 Vriksasana / Tree Pose

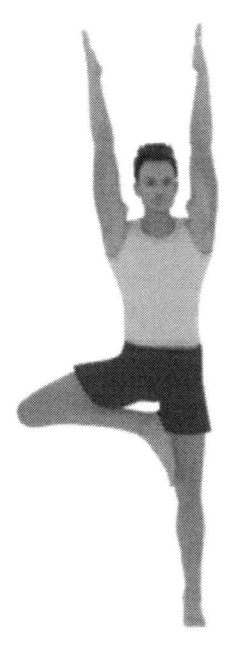

From Mountain pose, bend your left knee and shift your weight to the right leg. Point the left knee to the left by placing your heel on your right leg. Stare at one point on the floor. Now slide your left foot up as high as you can while still maintaining balance. Then, bring your hands together in prayer in front of your chest. Draw your shoulders back and stick your chest slightly out. Slowly bring your arms over your head into an "H" position. Breathe deeply and slowly. When you are done, exhale and go back to the mountain pose. Repeat on the other side.

Benefits: The tree pose builds strength in the ankles and knees. It also fosters balance, focus and memory.

Contraindications: Recent or chronic knee or hip injury.

Bharmanasana / Table position

Begin by kneeling down and put your hands on the floor. Make sure your knees are hip width apart, and place your feet directly behind your knees. Position your hands under the shoulders with your fingers facing in front of you. Keep your back flat and look down between your hands.

Benefits: Helps lengthen and realign the spine.

30 Makarasana / Dolphin pose

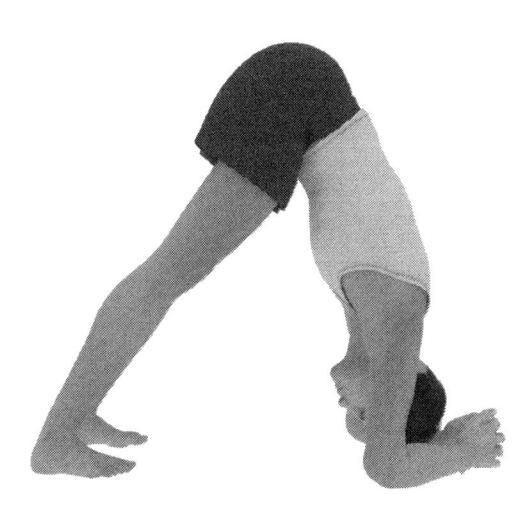

From downward-facing dog, slowly lower both forearms toward the ground with your shoulders over your elbows. Lift your upper back and place your head between your arms. Draw your shoulders together and down the spine.

Benefits: Lengthens the spine. Opens up the shoulders and upper back and builds upper body strength.

Contraindications: Injury to back, arm or shoulder.

30 Eka Pada Adho Mukha Svanasana / One legged downward facing dog

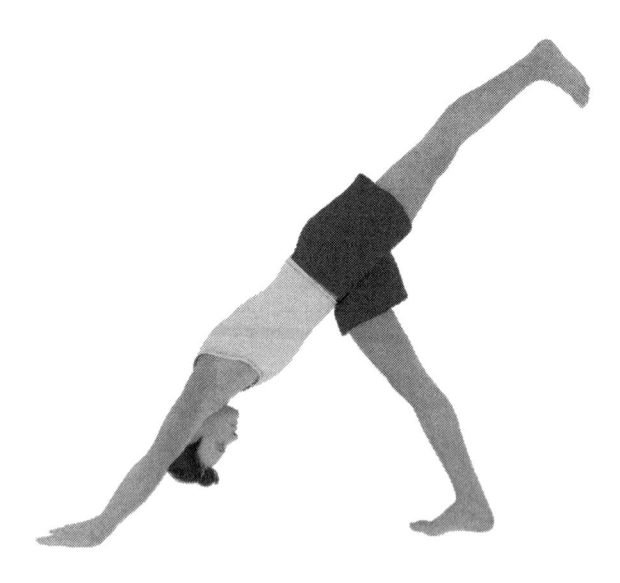

From downward-facing dog, extend one leg back and up as you bring the leg out of the hip. Take a few deep breaths and start over with the other leg.

Benefits: Deeper stretch in the hamstrings. Builds muscle in the extended leg.

Yoga Poses for cognitive benefits and psychological health

In general, practicing yoga will decrease stress, anxiety, and depression and give a huge boost to your mood and sense of wellbeing. But there are a few positions you can do to specifically target this area, as well as enhance your cognitive functioning and increase memory, mental clarity, and intelligence:

Ardha matsyendrasana / Half Spinal Twist

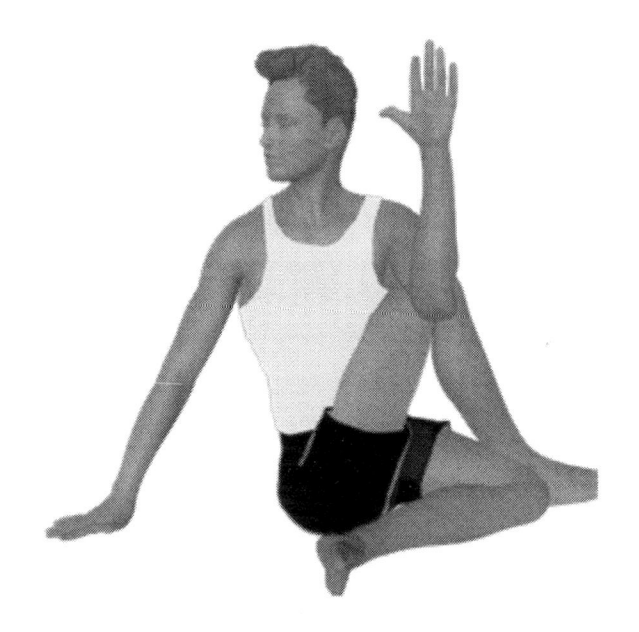

From a seated position, with the legs extended in front of the body, bend the right knee and place the right foot flat on the floor. Bend the left leg and bring the knee under the crook of the right leg, so that the left heel touches the right buttock. Bring the left arm to the right side of the body and to the other side of the right leg, and grasp the right ankle with the left hand. The right leg should be pressing against the left arm. Keeping the spine straight, exhale and twist your torso to the right, and press your right hand on the floor, elbow locked. Twist your neck to the right as far as is comfortable to add to the twisted position of this pose, but don't allow your shoulders to slouch. Keep your neck straight and upright.

The idea is to use your right leg and left arm to twist the spine without using the back muscles, so that the spine and back muscles are left to relax fully. You should not strain or force anything in this position. Breathe deeply for twenty counts of the breathe, then inhale and slowly return to the starting position.

Then repeat the whole position, this time on the left side.

Benefits: Half spinal twist relieves stress, anxiety, and depression. It helps release deep tension from the back, shoulders, and neck, which often accompanies stress. It is also an excellent back stretch that alternately stretches and contracts the muscles on each side of the back, and can improve back conditions such as slipped disc.

Vipareeta Karani Asana / Inverted Pose

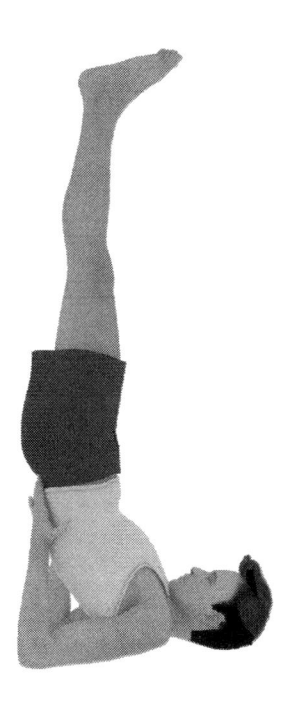

Lie flat on your back with your feet together. Your arms should be at your side, palms against the floor. Inhale while lying down.

Then, holding the breath, lift your legs towards the ceiling and bring them towards your head. Pressing down with your palms, letting the arms do the work, lift your buttocks from the floor, which will cause your back to bend. Lift up the palms but keep the elbows on the floor, then bring the palms against the lower part of your back just below the buttocks to support the weight. If that is too difficult, you can hold your palms against the buttocks. Your elbows and shoulders will support the weight of your body.

Keep your legs at a ninety-degree angle to the floor. Close your eyes and relax, breathing normally for as long as you are comfortable. Then, holding your breath again, bring the knees towards your head again, return your palms face-down to the floor, and slowly lower the buttocks to the floor, finally resting your legs and resuming the original position.

In the beginning, you may find it easier to prop your legs against the wall while holding this position.

Benefits: Inverted pose reverses the force of gravity on the body, which has a number of benefits. In particular, it causes blood flow to the head to increase. The increased blood flow in the brain benefits the mind, relieving anxiety, stress, and depression, improving cognitive functions, and increasing memory and intelligence. Inverted pose also relieves flatulence and hemorrhoids.

Yoga Poses for Meditation

Meditation is one of the most powerful tools for personal transformation out there. The following poses are designed specifically for meditation:

Sukhasana / *Comfortable Position*

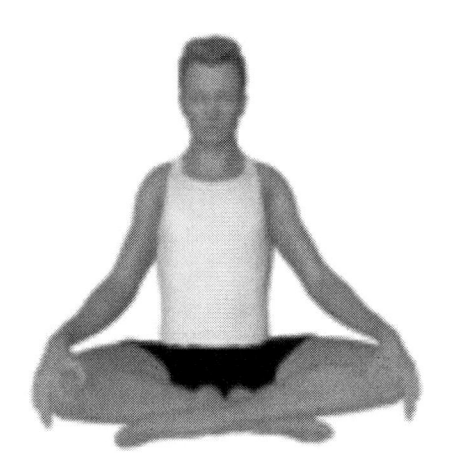

The easiest meditation position by far for beginners is *sukhasana* or the "comfortable pose." In this position, you cross your legs as you normally would when sitting on the floor. The spine and neck should be straight but relaxed, without any strain. Because of the position of the legs, this can be a little hard to achieve in *sukhasana*, so it will be much easier to keep your back straight if your butt is seated on a cushion two or three inches off the ground. Otherwise, if you can manage it, your back will feel more comfortable, and you will be able to keep your spine straight for longer periods of time, if you can sit in some of the more advanced meditation postures, such as the lotus position.

Your hands should rest in a *mudra* in which the forefinger rests on the inside of the thumb, forming a circle, and the other three fingers are extended but relaxed. The palms may face either up or down, resting on the knees, with the arms stretched forward and the elbows slightly bent.

Tilt your head slightly forward. You may keep your eyes either open or closed. If you hold your eyes open, allow them to rest on a point about four to five feet in front of you in empty space, your gaze relaxed and defocused.

Benefits: The main benefit of *sukhasana* is that it is easy to maintain for people whose bodies are unable to sit in the more difficult meditation positions. Otherwise, for longer periods of meditation, one of the other postures that allows the knees to touch the floor will yield much greater stability.

Padmasana / *Lotus Position*

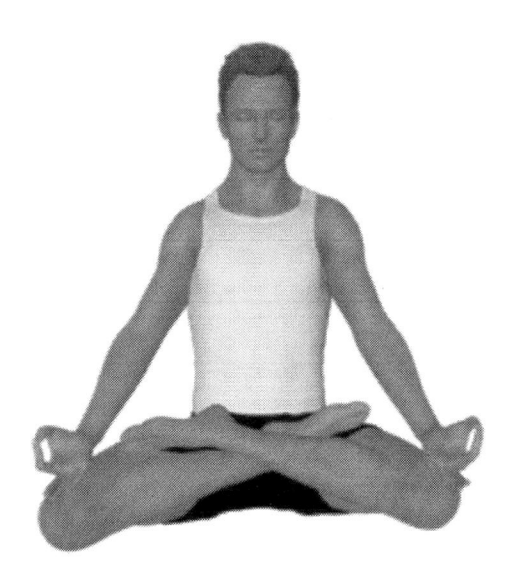

The *lotus position* is the classic and most famous meditation pose. If you can manage it, great. If you can't, don't sweat it. With *padmasana*, as with other yoga positions, it's very important not to force your body to do anything it doesn't want to do, or else you risk injuring yourself. So if you can't get yourself into the right position, simply practice the more dynamic poses from the health chapter and your flexibility will increase. In time, *padmasana* will be within reach for you. For now, if lotus position is just too much, try less demanding positions such as *sukhasana* and half-lotus.

This posture is famously hard to achieve for beginners and can cause pain on the legs, but if you are going to sit in meditation for long periods of time, it allows the highest level of stability and ease on the back. Moreover, the posture is especially good at allowing the body's *prana*, or subtle energy, to flow in a way that lends itself to deep and powerful meditative awareness.

To sit in the lotus position, sit cross-legged on the mat or cushion, with your left foot resting on the right thigh, and right foot resting on the left thigh. The back should be held straight but relaxed, with minimal effort and without tension, as if the spine were a stack of coins. The knees should touch the ground. The shoulders should be held somewhat back, like a vulture's wings, and the tongue rest at the roof of the mouth. The *mudra* or gesture of the hands may vary, but usually the hands rest, palms up, on the knees, with the nail of the forefinger touching the inside of the thumb.

Benefits: The lotus position allows for stability during long periods of sitting meditation. The posture not only allows a steady, sitting position without movement, it also encourages the mind to naturally calm down and rest in meditative awareness. Physically, this pose strengthens posture and spinal alignment, as well as improving digestion by allowing blood to flow to the digestive tract.

Contraindications: Do not attempt this posture if you have weak or injured knees. Also avoid it if you have great difficulty achieving it, or if sitting in *padmasana* causes physical pain. Before you attempt *padmasana*, it is good to practice other yoga positions that loosen the muscles and increase flexibility. If you suffer from sciatica, you should also avoid the lotus position.

Variations: In the variation called *ardha-padmasana* or half-lotus, one leg is drawn in and rests on the floor against the inside of the opposite thigh, while the other leg rests on top of the other thigh. This position is easier and requires less flexibility in the legs than the full lotus position.

Siddhasana / *Pose of the Masters*

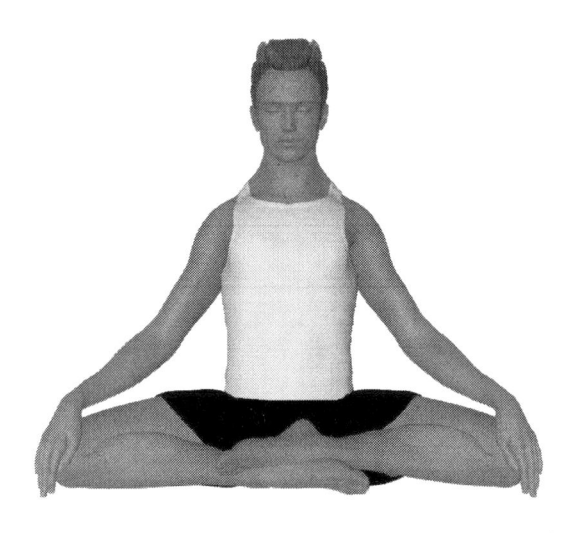

The right foot rests against the inside of the left thigh with the heel pressing against the perineum, so that this area is sitting on top of the right heel. Then the left leg is drawn in, with the left ankle resting on the right ankle. Tuck the toes of the left foot between the calf and thigh of the right leg. In the final position, the left feel should press into the pubic area above the genitals, so that the genitals are between the left and right heels.

There are two versions of this pose, one for women and one for men. The version for women is called *siddha yoni asana* and is much the same as described above, but with left and right reversed, with the *left* heel pressing against the labia, and the right foot on top, its heel pressing against the clitoris.

The hands and the rest of the body are held as in *sukhasana* and lotus position, described above.

Benefits: *Siddhasana* may allow for similar stability to the lotus position for those who aren't flexible enough to sit in full lotus. It benefits people who suffer from high blood pressure and prostate problems. It redirects the body's subtle energy upwards, away from the genitals. That means it decreases the sexual libido. I'll leave it up to you to decide whether or not that's a benefit!

How to Meditate

So now that we've gone over the different meditation positions, it will probably be useful if we actually talk a bit about *how* to meditate. Meditation is all the rage these days, with a lot of scientific research to back up its many benefits. It is not just used in therapy, but also in offices and at home to improve people's overall quality of life.

Meditation is proven to lower stress, increase concentration and cognitive performance, reduce anxiety and depression, and elevate your mood. The good news is, it's also easy to do, so if you have any doubt or hesitation about your ability to get into the practice, don't worry. Just try it out for five minutes.

Sit in one of the meditation positions described above, with your back straight but in a relaxed posture. You'll probably find that sitting on a cushion helps to decrease strain on your back and allow you to sit still for longer periods of time.

Your eyes may be open or closed. It's up to you. If you open your eyes, keep your gaze several feet in front of you and pointing downward, either resting on a point in space or on the floor. Either way, allow the eyes to relax, without any strain or strong focus.

Take a moment to feel the mass and weight of your body where you're sitting. Feel the pressure of your body pressing onto the floor or cushion, the weight of your feet or knees on the floor. Allow yourself to get a real sense of your body's weight where it comes into contact with the ground.

Then, take a couple of deep, heavy breaths—basically like sighing. This helps release any tension you're holding in your body. With your attention, scan the different parts of your body, trying to notice any tension or pain, or alternately any pleasurable sensation. You don't have to try to do anything with the tension, particularly, or try to change it. Just notice and acknowledge that it's there.

Now direct your attention to your breathing, to the in-and-out movements of your breath. Try to really feel the breath—the cold on your nostrils as you breathe in, the feeling of your lungs expanding, the diaphragm opening up. Feel the heat in your nose as you exhale, and the falling sensation of your chest as the breath leaves your body.

Don't try to concentrate in a tense way, but just allow the mind to rest on its object. The mind should melt into the breath and identify with it, in a relaxed way.

In the beginning, it helps to count the breath. So with each breath, count, *one, two, three*, etc., all the way up to *ten*. Then, start over again from *one*. If your mind wanders or you get distracted by thoughts or emotions, don't worry about it. Just gently return your mind to the breath, and gently resume counting again from one.

That's it! Sit like that, with your attention resting on the breath, for five to ten minutes. If you find yourself checking the time again and again, use an app on your phone to give you a chime when it's time to finish up your session, so that you can take your mind off the ticking of the clock.

Maintaining a consistent, daily meditation practice does wonders for your stress level and mood, giving you a happier, fuller experience of life. Just a short, five-minute meditation session in the morning sets the right mood for the rest of the day. Combined with the other yoga positions discussed in this book, meditation is a powerful way of increasing your overall wellbeing and quality of life.

The Benefits of Yoga

Over the past decade or so, a vast amount of scientific research has been carried out to investigate the benefits of Yoga for the human mind and body. The National Institute of Health has spent millions of dollars toward research on yoga, and nowadays it seems like new studies claiming new benefits of yoga are emerging every single day.

Thousands of peer-reviewed studies now been conducted on the benefits of yoga and the truth is practicing yoga has so many benefits that I could not possibly list them all in this book. So here are a few noteworthy benefits of developing a consistent yoga practice:

- Improves flexibility
- Builds muscle strength
- Reduces risk of heart disease and stroke
- Eases Asthma
- Improves memory
- Reduces insomnia
- Relieves pain more effectively than medication
- Perfects posture
- Lowers blood sugar
- Prevents cartilage and joint breakdown
- Protects spine
- Helps with weight loss
- Slows down the aging process
- Helps recover from addiction
- Helps beat depression
- Increases energy levels
- Increases endurance
- Enhances fertility

- Reduces pain associated with arthritis, fibromyalgia and other chronic conditions
- Boosts immune system functionality
- Increases blood flow
- Reduces stress and anxiety
- Improves relationships
- Improves athletic performance
- Lowers blood pressure more effectively than medication
- Regulates adrenal glands
- Improves focus
- Cultivates mental strength
- Fosters creativity
- Helps sleep deeper
- Decreases muscle tension
- Improves balance
- Enhances feelings of happiness and vitality
- Enhances self-awareness
- Fosters peace of mind, happiness and joy
- Develops intuition
- Builds wisdom

Turning Yoga into a habit

Yoga is very much like going to the gym. Practice it regularly, and you become fit. Slack off, on the other hand, and you become chubby. In order to attain profound levels of inner peace, mental clarity, and happiness, you must practice yoga consistently.

In 2010, a study conducted at University College London showed that it takes on average 66 days to build a new habit. This means you need to invest about two months of effort before the behavior of meditation becomes automatic – something that you do without even thinking about it – a habit.

The key to making yoga automatic is to make it your top priority for the next 66 days. Yoga essentially has to become the most important activity in your day. Here are 9 ways to turn yoga into a habit:

Work on Your WHY
It's important to get crystal clear on why you want to make yoga a habit. Go through the list of benefits of yoga again and decide exactly why you want to practice yoga. Are you motivated to relieve stress, crush anxiety, or build a stronger body? Make sure your WHY resonates deeply within you. When you have figured out your WHY, start visualizing your success. Imagine how your life will be when you achieve your goal and use this image as fuel and motivation to keep you going throughout your yoga journey.

Commit to the activity
Take a moment and make an oath to yourself to start doing yoga every single day from now on. Firmly set your intention that you are going to do this and never give up. Feel the energy rising inside your body and seal the commitment with your heart.

Start Small

There is no "right" amount of time to do yoga for. If you're a beginner, don't fall into the trap of trying to do yoga for hours on end. Your simply aren't trained to sustain it yet. You can start with as little as 5 minutes of daily yoga and you can gradually build your way up from there. The key is to not overwhelm yourself when you're starting out– 5 minutes of yoga everyday is much better than 5 hours of punctual yoga.

Decide on a fixed time and a trigger

When you are trying to develop a new habit, it's very important to have a trigger that reminds you to perform the new behavior around the same time everyday. The easiest way is to incorporate your meditation into your morning routine or evening routine. The key is to choose a trigger that makes it easy to juxtapose the new behavior onto an already existing habit. You can decide for example that you are going to meditate everyday day right after you brush your teeth in the morning or right before you go to bed.

Track Your Progress

Use a calendar to track your progress and make it visible. Mark down every time you follow through on your new habit. This will inspire you to keep going even when things get difficult. It will suddenly become more painful to break your streak. You can also use habit-tracking apps, which I have found to be extremely useful.

Be Accountable

Find an accountability buddy, preferably someone who is also looking to develop a long-term meditation practice. This will greatly increase your chances of success. When you have someone that holds you accountable, you will find it much more difficult to miss a session.

Split your sessions

One simple trick you can utilize to make your meditation more enjoyable is to split your meditation into two smaller sessions. This will allow you to easily increase your overall session length. Instead of trying to sit for a whole 30 minutes for example, it is much easier sit for 15 minutes in the morning and 15 minutes in the evening.

Reward Yourself

Whatever gets rewarded gets repeated. Your brain is constantly associating pain and pleasure to everything you do. So if you want your meditation habit to stick, trick your brain by rewarding yourself right after you have completed your meditation. It can be something as simple as giving yourself a pat on the back and saying to yourself: " Good job, you made progress today!".

Remember, consistent action is the only way to make mediation a habit. By practicing it everyday, you will create new neural pathways that will make the behavior automatic and you soon enough you won't even have to expand any willpower to sit down and meditate. Make meditation a long-term habit and it will transform every aspect of your life.

Conclusion

I hope this book was able to help you understand how practicing yoga can bring strength, happiness and peace into your life. The next step is to apply what you have learned and develop a long-term yoga practice. It can be a challenging process but I assure you that it is well worth it - You will enjoy a happier, more peaceful and balanced life free from stress, anxiety, and depression.

I wish you success on your yoga journey and I hope you quickly start reaping the amazing benefits that yoga has to offer.

Finally, if you enjoyed this book, then I'd like to ask you a favor. Would you be kind enough to share your thoughts and post a review of this book on Amazon?

Your voice is important for this book to reach as many people as possible. The more reviews this book gets, the more people will be able to find it and enjoy the incredible benefits of yoga.

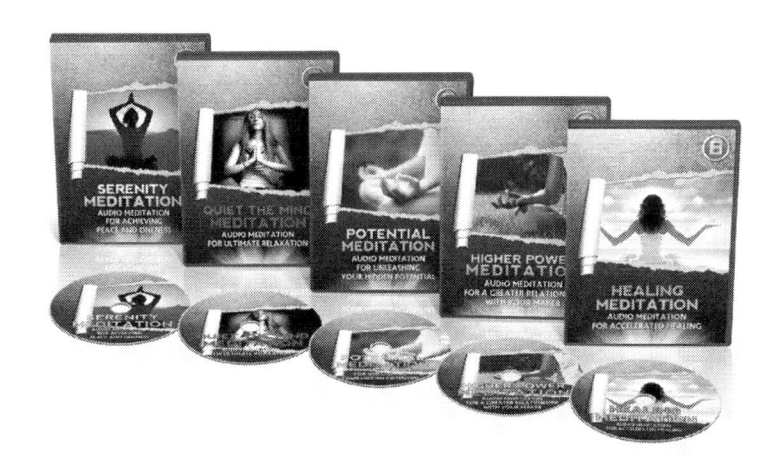

Bonus: Free Guided Meditation Series (5 Audiobooks)

→ Go to http://www.projectlimitlesslife.com/bonus-2/ to get your FREE Guided Meditation Series

You will get immediate access to:

- Healing Audio Meditation
- Higher Power Audio Meditation
- Potential Audio Meditation
- Quiet the Mind Audio Meditation
- Serenity Audio Meditation

You will also join my private kindle club and be the first to know about my upcoming kindle books!

Preview of
The Meditation Beginner's Bible

Introduction

From the outside meditation can seem like an esoteric, mystical endeavor exclusively reserved to enlightened monks and spiritual adepts. This could not be further from the truth. Meditation is not only accessible to anyone, it is extremely easy to learn and the benefits are only a few minutes away. In fact, a study by Dr Fadel Zeidan at Wake Forest Medical Center has shown only 80 minutes of meditation to be more effective for pain relief than even morphine.

In this book you will learn exactly why many highly successful people like Russell Simons, Arianna Huffington, Oprah Winfrey and Hugh Jackman set aside time off their busy schedules to engage in the life-changing practice of meditation.

Meditation can seem a bit daunting at first, especially if, like most of us, you're always up in your head, constantly dwelling on the past and worrying about the future. However, the moment you recognize that meditation is not about trying to empty your mind, but rather about observing your thoughts as they come and go without energizing them, you begin to awaken and meditation becomes the most blissful, transformative moment of the day.

This book will show you how to instill simple meditation techniques into your daily routine, inevitably leading you to a more successful, happier and healthier life.

Chapter 1 - What is meditation?

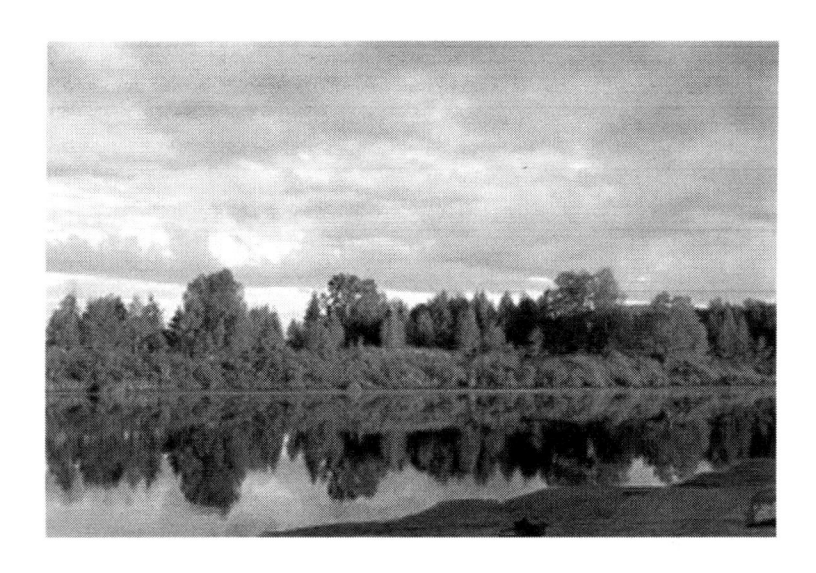

"The gift of learning to meditate is the greatest gift you can give yourself in this lifetime."
Sogyal Rinpoche

The word meditation and the word medicine come from the same Latin root "medicus" which means to cure. In the same way medicine cures sickness that exists inside the physical body by restoring it to a healthy state, meditation cures sickness that exists within the mind by returning it to its natural state of peace, joy and happiness.

But how does the mind become sick? Well, in our modern society most of us suffer from what we call compulsive thinking. We have this inner voice that is constantly thinking, ruminating the past, worrying about the future, and hence we never fully experience the present moment.
Take a few seconds right now and become aware of your breathing. Observe the changing sensations of your breath as

you inhale and then exhale. Be aware of your lungs filling and emptying themselves. Become one with your breath and notice the subtle gap between your incoming and outcoming breath - let yourself completely dissolve into the activity of breathing.

If you did this little exercise, I bet you noticed your mind becoming a bit more still. When you rest your attention on your breath, you effectively step away from the chaotic impulses of the mind and you connect to your true Self – that eternal part of you that is beyond the ephemeral, ever-wavering physical realm.

Meditation is essentially a vehicle for accessing a higher level of consciousness that is beyond thought, where you are reconnected to your deepest self, your true nature of joy, peace and happiness. When you meditate, you effectively increase your level of self-awareness and you awaken to the things that are beyond thought - love, beauty, peace... This cannot be rationalized intellectually; however it can be experienced when you bring stillness into your mind.

Moreover, meditation does not require effort. As mentioned earlier, it is not about trying to empty your mind. Spiritual leader Deepak Chopra puts it beautifully: "*Meditation is not a way of making your mind quiet. It is a way of entering into the quiet that is already there - buried under the 50 000 thoughts the average person thinks everyday.*"

When you practice meditation, you gain control over your mind, you break the cycle of seeking stimulation from the external world and you learn to draw your state from within. Meditation is truly a transformative experience that can have profound effects not just on your mind, but on virtually every aspect of your life – your body, relationships, health and even your career.

Chapter 2 - The Benefits of Meditation

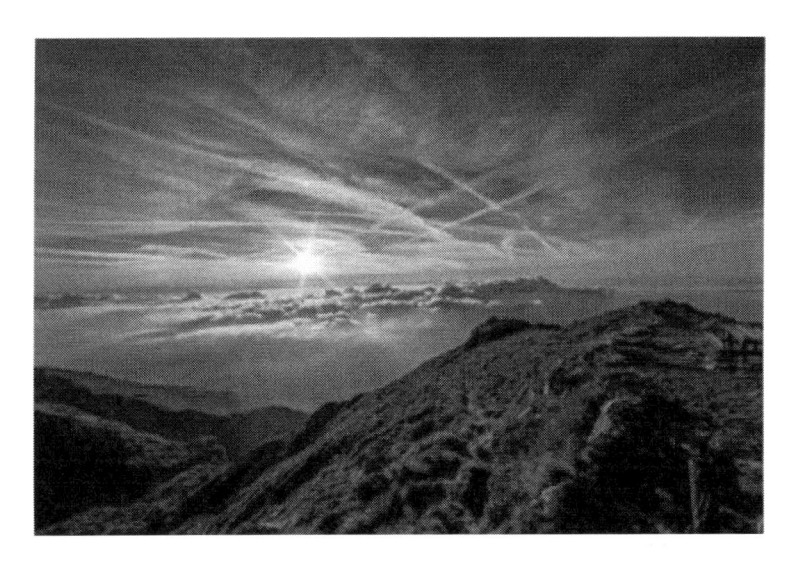

"Meditation more than anything in my life was the biggest ingredient of whatever success I've had."
Ray Dalio

Over the past decade, a vast amount of scientific research has been carried out to investigate the benefits of meditation for the human mind and body. The National Institute of Health has spent over $100 million toward research on meditation, and nowadays it seems like new studies professing the benefits of meditation are emerging everyday.

As a result of the various scientific discoveries on the benefits of meditation, a growing number of hospitals and medical centers are now teaching meditation to patients in order to address various health ailments, relieve pain and fight stress. For example, one famous meditation program called *Mindfulness Based Stress Reduction*, which was created in 1979 by Dr Jon Kabat-Zinn has become so popular that it is now offered in over 200 medical centers around the world.

One remarkable example of the effectiveness of meditation for pain relief is shown in a study conducted by Dr Fadel Zeidan at the Wake Forest Medical Center in North Carolina. In the study, 15 people who had never practiced meditation attended four, 20-minute mindfulness meditation classes. The participants' brain activity was examined before and after the training using magnetic resonance imaging. During both scans, they were exposed to a pain-inducing heat device. The results were impressive: After the training, the participant's pain intensity was reduced by about 40% and their pain unpleasantness by around 57%: 80 minutes of meditation was more effective than pain relieving drugs like morphine, which normally reduces pain by about 25%.

Meditation has also become popular in the corporate world, with some leading companies like Google providing meditation classes to their employees to relieve stress, improve focus and boost productivity. The search giant even took it a step further by building a labyrinth to encourage the practice of walking meditation. Moreover, Google is not the only company that is embracing meditation. In fact, other big corporations like Apple, Nike, Yahoo, McKinsey & Co... have all brought meditation to their workplaces in an endeavor to keep employees happy and productive.

Even schools are now adopting meditation to make kids calmer and more focused. Youth meditation program are being installed everywhere in the US, England, Canada and India. In 2014, Educational Psychology Review examined 15 peer-reviewed studies on meditation in schools and concluded that the practice had a myriad of positive effects on students, such as lessened anxiety, increased focus and stronger friendships.

Over 3,000 scientific studies have now been conducted on the benefits of meditation and the truth is practicing meditation has so many benefits that I could not list them all in this book. So here are 53 noteworthy benefits of developing a regular meditation practice:

Health Benefits

- Lowers blood pressure more effectively than medication
- Relieves pain more effectively than morphine
- Slows the progression of HIV
- Helps prevent fibromyalgia and arthritis
- Reduces risk of Alzheimer's
- Reduces risk of heart disease and stroke
- Provides rest deeper than sleep
- Helps recover from addiction
- Improves cardiovascular function
- Relieves irritable bowel syndrome
- Increases energy levels
- Slows down the aging process
- Improves athletic performance
- Improves quality of sleep
- Improves fertility
- Decreases muscle tension
- Improves skin tone
- Increases air flow to the lungs
- Boosts the immune system
- Reduces inflammation

Mental and Emotional Benefits

- Improves attention, focus and ability to work under pressure
- Helps manage ADHD
- Improves intelligence and memory
- Improves critical thinking and decision-making
- Fosters creativity
- Slows down cognitive decline
- Builds composure and calm in all situations
- Increases brain connectivity
- Improves mental strength
- Improves sex life
- Cultivates willpower
- Boosts cognitive function
- Increases grey matter in the hippocampus and frontal areas of the brain
- Helps manage emotional eating
- Promotes good mood
- Improves working memory and executive functioning
- Helps beat depression
- Reduces stress and anxiety
- Improves emotional stability
- Fosters empathy and positive relationships
- Decreases feelings of nervousness
- Reduces social isolation
- Enhances feelings of happiness and vitality
- Improves communication with other people
- Develops a sense of calm and serenity

Spiritual Benefits

- Enhances self-awareness
- Fosters peace of mind, happiness and joy
- Increases self-acceptance
- Boosts self-compassion
- Increases self-esteem
- Develops intuition
- Builds wisdom
- Increases capacity for love

→ Available on Amazon

Preview of
The Mindfulness Beginner's Bible

Chapter 1 - What is mindfulness?

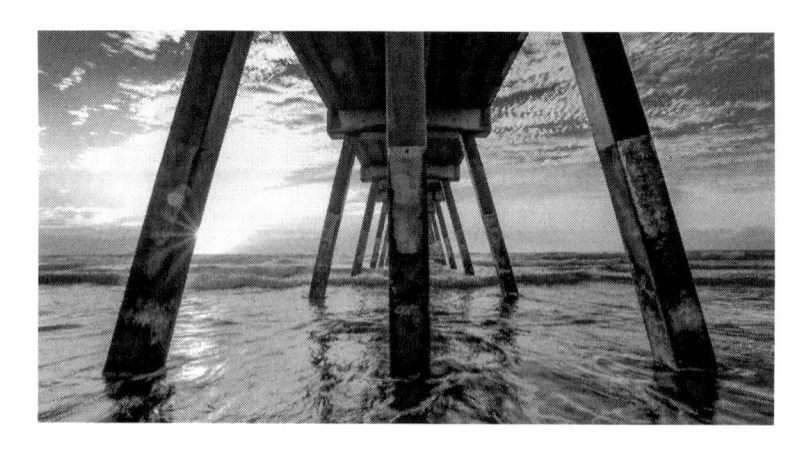

"Life is a dance. Mindfulness is witnessing that dance."
Amit Ray

Have you ever started eating a packet of chips and then suddenly realize that there is nothing left? This is one example of mindlessness that most of us experience on a daily basis. We, as humans often get so absorbed in our thoughts that we fail to experience what is happening right in front of us.

In modern society, most of us suffer from a condition called compulsive thinking. We have this hysterical inner voice that is constantly jumping from one thought to the next, obsessing about every little detail that could go wrong, complaining, comparing and criticizing everything and everyone. Sadly, most of us have become hostages to the whims of our minds, to the point where we even identify with the mind, thinking that we are our thoughts, when in reality we are the awareness behind our thoughts.

The moment you start observing your thoughts without identifying with them, you enter a higher level of consciousness beyond the mind and you reconnect with your true Self – the eternal part of you that is beyond the transient, ever-wavering physical realm.

Take a few seconds right now and become mindful of your hands. Feel the warmth that emanates from them. Rest your attention on every sensation in your hands. Feel your blood pulsing through them. Become one with your hands and notice the subtle tingling sensation as you become aware of them.

If you did this little exercise, I bet you noticed your mind becoming a bit more still. When you rest your attention on your body, you are living actively in the now. Awareness of the body instantly grounds you in the present moment and helps you awaken to a vast realm of consciousness beyond the mind, where all the things that truly matter - love, beauty, peace, creativity and joy - arise from.

Research has shown that we spend up to 50% of the time inside our heads - a state of mindlessness where we are continuously consumed by the chaotic impulses of our minds that are constantly thinking, ruminating the past and worrying about the future. Sadly, most people go through life in a walking haze, never really experiencing the present moment, which is our most precious asset.

Mindfulness is about being fully immersed into your inner and outer experience of the present moment. One of the best definitions of mindfulness is provided by the mindfulness teacher Jon Kabat-Zinn: "*Mindfulness means paying attention in a particular way; On purpose, in the present moment, and non-judgmentally.*"

Jon Kabat-Zinn breaks down mindfulness into its fundamental components: In mindfulness, our attention is held...

On purpose
Paying attention on purpose means intentionally directing your awareness. It goes beyond merely being aware of something. It means deliberately focusing your conscious awareness wherever you choose to, instead of being carried away in the perpetual storm of your thoughts.

Secondly, our attention is plunged...

In the Present Moment
The mind's natural tendency is to wander away from the present and get lost in the past or the future. Mindfulness requires being in complete non-resistance to the present moment.

Finally, our attention is held...

Non judgmentally
In mindfulness there is no judgment, there is no labeling, there is no resistance and there is no attachment. You simply observe your thoughts, feelings and sensations as they arise without ever energizing with them. As soon as you realize that you are not your thoughts, but the observer behind your thoughts, they will immediately lose power over your.

Mindfulness goes beyond basic awareness of your present experience. You could be aware that you are drinking tea, for example, however mindfully drinking tea looks very different. When you are mindfully drinking tea, you are purposefully aware of the entire process of drinking tea – you feel the warmth of the cup, the subtleties in smell and taste of the tea, the sensation of heat as you press your lips against the cup... – you intentionally immerse yourself in every single sensory detail that makes up the experience of drinking tea, to the point where you completely dissolve into the activity.

Mindfulness is about maintaining the intention of being completely plunged into your experience, whether it is drinking tea, breathing or doing the dishes. You can bring mindfulness to virtually any activity in your life.

Chapter 2 - The Power of the Present Moment

"I have realized that the past and future are real illusions, that they exist in the present, which is what there is and all there is."
Alan Watts

When you think about it, the present moment is the only moment that really exists. The past and the future are merely persistent illusions – the past is obviously over, and the future hasn't happened yet. As the saying goes, *"Tomorrow never comes"*. The future is merely a mental construct that is always around the corner.

Even when you dwell on the past or worry about the future, you're doing so in the present moment. At the end of the day, the present moment is all you and I have, and to spend most of our time outside the present means we are never truly living. Spiritual leader Eckhart Tolle puts it beautifully: *"People don't realize that now is all there ever is; there is no past or future except as memory or anticipation in your mind."*

However, most people spend most of their waking time imprisoned within the walls of their own thoughts, usually in regret of the past or in fear of the future, which are two ways of not living at all.

The present is the only moment in our lives where we have complete control over our destiny. We can decide our course of action only in the now – we can make a new friend, start a new business, get back to the gym, decide to stop smoking... The present is the only moment where your creative power can be exercised; it is the only place where you have full control over your life. Embracing the present moment is the only way to live a happier, healthier and more fulfilling life. As Buddha said, *"The secret of health for both mind and body is not to mourn for the past, worry about the future, or anticipate troubles, but to live in the present moment wisely and earnestly."*

The biggest obstacle that keeps us from living in the present moment is the mind. Embracing mindfulness is a journey that requires practice and dedication, but it is a process that will inevitably lead you to a much happier and more fulfilling life where every moment is lived to the fullest. Here are 8 steps to start living in the present moment:

Practice non-resistance

The first step towards living in the present is learning to live in acceptance. You must learn to accept your life as it is today, rather than wish it was any other way. You must come into complete non-resistance with your current experience of life. By letting go of the hold the past has over you, you free your mind from unproductive thoughts and you reclaim the present moment. As Eckhart Tolle says, *"Accept - then act. Whatever the present moment contains, accept it as if you had chosen it. Always work with it, not against it."*

Focus on the Now

In order to live in the present moment, you must focus on what you are doing in the now, whatever it may be. If you are doing the dishes, then do the dishes. If you're eating dinner, then eat dinner. Don't view the seemingly mundane activities in your life as nuisances that you hurry to get out of the way. These moments are what our lives are made up of, and not being present in them means we are not truly living.

Don't take your thoughts too seriously

Identification with the mind is the root of much unhappiness, disease and misery in the world. Most people have become so identified with their mental chatter that they become slaves to their own compulsive thoughts. Being unable to stop thinking and means we are never living in the present moment. When you learn to observe your thoughts as they come and go without identification, you step away from the chaotic impulses of the mind and you ground yourself in the now.

Meditate

You don't have to meditate to be mindful, but research has shown that engaging in a regular meditation practice has a spillover effect on the rest of your life. When you meditate you essentially carry the state of stillness and awareness that you experience during your meditation session into the rest of your day. Meditation is practice for the rest of your life.

Pay attention to the little things

Notice the seemingly insignificant things around you. Pay attention to nature for example. Notice the greenery around you - be grateful for every tree, every plant, every flower and realize that you could not survive without their presence. Go through your life as if everything is a miracle. From the majestic rising of the sun, to the chirping of birds outside your window, to the fact that your heart is beating every single second – life is truly a miracle to behold when you immerse yourself in the present moment.

Do one thing at a time

Multitasking is the opposite of living in the now. When your attention is divided between several tasks like eating, driving, making a phone call, you cannot fully experience the present moment. Studies have shown that people who multitask take about 50% longer to complete a task with a 50% larger error rate. To be more mindful, you must become a single-tasker. When you're eating, just eat. When you're talking to people, just talk to them. Develop the habit of being completely immersed into whatever you're doing. Not only will you be more efficient, but you'll also be more alive.

Don' try to quiet your mind

Living in the present moment does not require any special effort. The present moment is already at your fingertips. There is no need to expand energy to empty your mind. In mindfulness there is no stress, no struggle and no effort because you are not trying to force anything – you are in complete non-resistance to your current experience of life.

Stop worrying about the future

Worry takes you out of the present moment and in the future into an infinite world of possibilities. You cannot worry about the future and simultaneously live in the present moment. Instead of worrying about things that may or may not happen, spend you time preparing to the best of your ability and let go of the rest. Worrying won't change the future, but it will definitely elevate the cortisol levels in your body and drain you of your vital energy.

Printed in Great Britain
by Amazon